NATURAL KILLER CELLS: THE FUTURE OF CANCER IMMUNOTHERAPY

An overview of how natural killer cells can be genetically engineered to fight tumors

Priyanka Senthil

ISBN-13: 9798593219954

Cover design by: Art Painter
Cover Image by: Creative Commons (CC BY 2.0)
Library of Congress Control Number: 2018675309
Printed in the United States of America

I dedicate this book to my parents, my teachers, and researchers/doctors who help to advance science and technology for the benefit of our society.

CONTENTS

PREFACE

This book explains the promising role of Natural Killer cell in cancer immunotherapy and the potential challenges that need to be overcome.

NK CELLS: A CLOSER LOOK

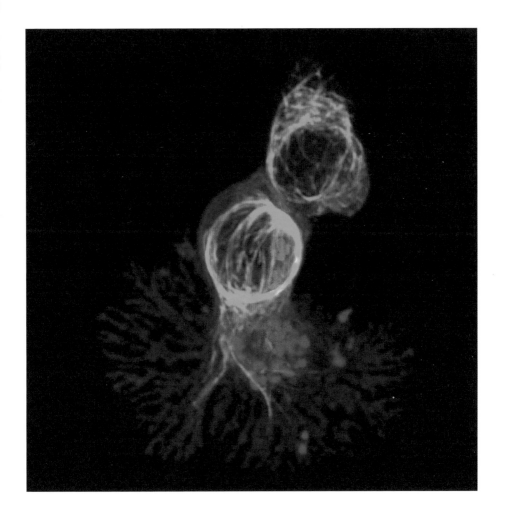

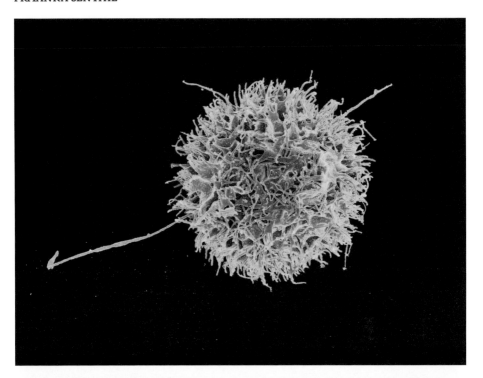

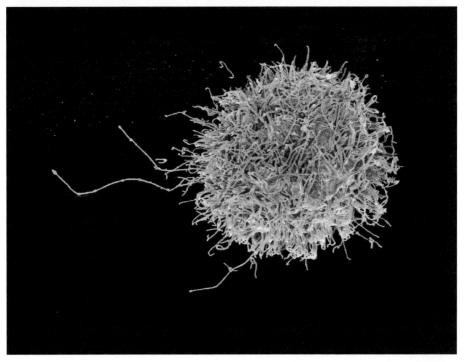

THE FIELD OF CANCER IMMUNOTHERAPY

Cancer has been one of the very few diseases that has proved to be difficult to cure despite our scientific and technological advancements. Even after investing billions of dollars in research, we have not found a definite cure for a disease that affects more than 17 million people worldwide. Why is it so difficult to cure cancer?

Cancer develops when normal cells accumulate harmful mutations. Most cells can detect these mutations and fix them or undergo apoptosis (programmed cell death) to avoid harming other cells. However, in cancerous cells, these mutations are ignored, and the cells grow without limits. The cancerous cells then invade other tissues and organs.

There are more than 100 types of cancers and once a cancer becomes metastasized, it becomes very hard to cure.

Many aggressive tumors will have multiple populations of slightly different cancerous cells. Different mutations can arise, giving way to several different subclones. This makes therapy even harder since a treatment that works for one subclone, might not work for another subclone.

Tumors can also manipulate the body to feed it blood by redirecting blood vessels to the tumor site and by tricking the immune system to think the tumor is not harmful.

Cancerous cells are also able to easily adapt to their environment and can change their molecular and cellular characteristics if put under stress (like during radiation or chemotherapy).

Traditionally, we've treated cancer with radiation, chemotherapy, or surgery to remove tumors. However, a new strategy has developed recently. Instead of killing the cancer cells by external treatments, this strategy is dependent on training the immune system to attack the cancer itself. This is called immunotherapy.

This book is centered around cancer immunotherapy. Therefore, it is important to first understand what immunotherapy is. Simply put, immunotherapy is using your body's own immune system to fight cancer. There are several different methods that use this framework. For example, we can stimulate our own immune system and prime it so that it recognizes cancer and determines the best response to fight it. We can also introduce parts of the immune system like proteins and antibodies into the body to help the immune system fight cancer.

Therefore, we can use what we know about our immune system to keep foreign substances out. Though there have been decades of research in this field, it was not until a few years ago that proven and tested treatments for melanoma were created. Now there are more than 900 studies in the field of immunotherapy.

Immunotherapy has changed the way we view our immune system. Instead of using external treatments, we train our own immune system to recognize foreign substances and use its innate ability to fight them. The idea is that if our body can recognize potential dangers in the earlier stages, then our immune system has a higher likelihood of being able to defend itself.

Cancerous cells are able to rapidly replicate and grow because they block checkpoint inhibitors that help to keep the replication of normal cells in check. We're starting to learn how we can manipulate the inhibitors that block these checkpoint inhibitors in cancerous cells to prevent their growth and improve survival.

One of the most recent advancements is joint therapy, which is the integration of immunotherapy and chemotherapy. Joint therapy has been shown to be extremely effective, especially in a sample of patients with metastasized lung cancer. This type of therapy has more than doubled the cancer response rate when compared to its rate with chemotherapy alone.

However, we are still in the infancy stages of treating patients with immunotherapy. The future for immunotherapy is further, more active combination regiments in which you have 2 or even 3 immune therapies that activate the immune system and attack the tumor in different ways, working synergistically together in order to get more prolonged responses that could even turn into cures for patients with melanoma and other tumor types as well.

New immunotherapeutic targets are being discovered nearly every day, increasing our hope that effective therapies will soon become available for all tumor profiles. We have just discovered the tip of the iceberg. There is still much more to explore.

INTRODUCTION

T cells, which are lymphocyte immune cells, have largely been used in the past in therapeutic approaches against Leukemia.

However, a new type of immune cell called the chimeric antigen receptor-modified natural killer (CAR NK) cell is stealing the spotlight. CAR NK cells are able to fight against many different types of tumors and hematological malignancies. They work in a similar manner to T cells, but they need to be genetically modified to express CARs in NK cells, which will provide them with the ability to target specific tumor types. CAR NK cells have shown to have many advantages when compared to T cells in immunotherapy because they can be engineered to target a wider range of tumors, are quicker to produce, safer since they reduce the risk of graft-versus-host disease (GVHD), and are cheaper.

This book discusses various studies on CAR NK cells, the development and potential applications of these cells, and the advantages and disadvantages of a CAR NK cell-mediated immunotherapy.

BACKGROUND

It is estimated that around 606,520 people will die from cancer in 2020 in US alone. Though there are new chemotherapeutic drugs, radiotherapy, and innovative surgical techniques, there is no definite cure for malignant tumors. Therefore, to reduce death rates, potential treatment modalities are being investigated.

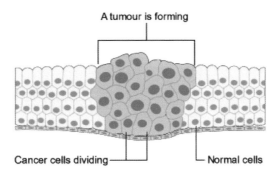

Figure-1: Diagram showing how cancer cells keep on reproducing to form a tumor.
Credit: Cancer Research UK / Wikimedia Commons

One of the most promising treatments is immunotherapy. But the idea of immunotherapy is not new. It was first proposed back in 1891 when a surgical oncologist, William Coley, suggested that the body's immune system can be enhanced to attack tumors. Coley injected over 1000 cancer patients with heat-killed streptococcal organisms to cause erysipelas (a bacterial skin infection) to stimulate the body's "resisting powers." Sometimes it worked, but often it did not. As a result, during the 20th century, surgery, radiation, and chemotherapy were the main forms of cancer treatment. With the aid of advanced scientific technologies, in the 21st century, scientists were able to discover that the body's immune system has "checkpoints" to protect the body from attacking its own cells. Cancer cells are able to manipulate this system by expressing proteins that would activate these checkpoints. Scientists made a major breakthrough when they discovered a protein called CTLA-4 that had checkpoint-like effects. By blocking the CTLA-4 protein using a monoclonal antibody called Ipilimumab (checkpoint inhibitor), scientists found that the body was able to fight tumors. The evolution of checkpoint inhibitors has led to the development of other immunotherapy treatments such as chimeric antigen receptor T cell (CAR-T) therapy. In CAR-T cell therapy, patients' T cells are genetically modified to add receptors that can search and kill cancer cells that express specific proteins. CAR-T cell therapy proved to be effective in patients who had developed tumors in many parts of their bodies.

However, CAR-T cell treatment is not perfect; it has several side effects, including flu-like symptoms, mild nausea, and sometimes life-threatening inflammation. Also, CAR-T cells can only attack cancer cells that express the specific proteins they are genetically engineered to identify. Additionally, one of the major hardships with the generation of an autologous CAR-T cell product, which is derived from the patient, is that it is too cumbersome and restrictive for widespread clinical use. In fact, it takes a minimum of two to three weeks to manufacture CAR-T cells. Therefore, for a patient in critical condition with a rapidly advancing disease, treatment with CAR-T cells would be an impractical choice. Additionally, it is difficult to collect the number of lymphocytes needed to allow for the successful generation of CAR-T cells. Furthermore, allogeneic T cells, which are transported from a donor, can cause graft-versus-host disease (GVHD), a condition that occurs when the donor's T cells (the graft) attack the recipient's healthy cells (the host) thinking they are foreign. GVHD can occur any time after transplant and can range from mild to severe, though most cases are life-threatening.

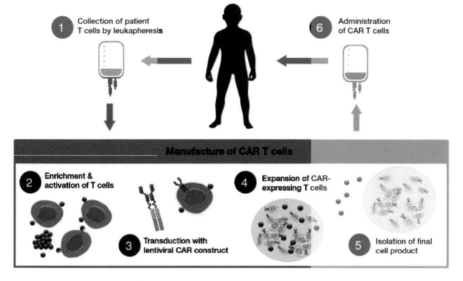

Figure-2: Diagram of CAR-T cell treatment process. The treatment process for patients receiving CAR-T cell therapy begins with leukapheresis of the patient's T cells. Once isolated, autologous T cells are sent for manufacturing to produce genetically modified CAR-T cells, which are reprogrammed to facilitate targeted killing of CD19+ B cells. The treatment process is completed with intravenous infusion of CAR-T cells back to the patient. CAR chimeric antigen receptor.

Credit: Hucks, George & Rheingold, Susan / Blood Cancer Journal

The newly discovered chimeric antigen receptor-modified natural killer (CAR-NK) cells are more promising than CAR-T cells. NK cells are cytotoxic (cell-killing) and kill their targets in a non-specific manner. This means that NK cells do not have to recognize a specific antigen on viral-infected cells or cancer cells.[1],[2] This enhances their immunosurveillance.

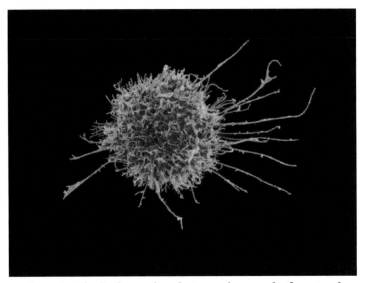

**Figure-3: Colorized scanning electron micrograph of a natural
killer cell from a human donor.**
Credit: NIAID / Flickr

The NK cells decide whether or not to kill cells based on signals from activating receptors and inhibitory receptors on the
NK cell surface. Activating receptors 'switch on' the NK cell
when they recognize molecules expressed on the surface of cancer cells. Similarly, inhibitory receptors 'switch off' the NK cell.
When they recognize cognate major histocompatibility complex class I (MHC I) receptors expressed on the surface of normal
healthy cells, killing is prevented. The genes that compose the
MHC encode surface proteins that are expressed on cells. MHC
class I molecules present endogenous antigens, while MHC class
II molecules present exogenous antigens, thereby helping the NK
cells distinguish host cells from unknown cells. Cancer cells and
infected cells become vulnerable to NK cell killing because they
often lose their MHC I. Once the decision to kill is made, cytotoxic granules are released by the NK cell, leading to lysis of
the target cell. Unlike a CAR-T cell, a CAR-NK cell does not carry
the risk of GVHD, and opens the doors for development of off-
the-shelf allogeneic products that could be readily available for

immediate clinical use.[3],[4] Furthermore, since CAR-NK cells have the ability to retain their full array of native receptors, they have a natural ability to identify and target cancer cells, which could omit the risk of relapse due to a loss of CAR-targeted antigen, as noted in CAR-T treatments.[5] This would ultimately make disease escape through downregulation of the CAR target antigen less likely.

NK CELL ACTIVATION/ DEACTIVATION AND KILLING MECHANISM

NK cells are called "natural" killers because they have the ability to kill cancer and virus-infected cells without prior sensitization, which is crucial for cancer immunotherapy. NK cells are primarily found in the blood, liver, and spleen, but can also be found in lymph nodes.[6],[7]

As described earlier, almost all NK cell functions - degranulation, cytokine release, and cytotoxicity - are governed by signals from activating receptors and inhibitory receptors. The main activating receptors include natural cytotoxicity receptors (NCRs) and C-type lectin-like activating immunoreceptors (NKG2D)[2], while the main inhibitory receptors include killer Ig-like receptors (KIRs) and heterodimeric C-type lectin receptors (NKG2A).

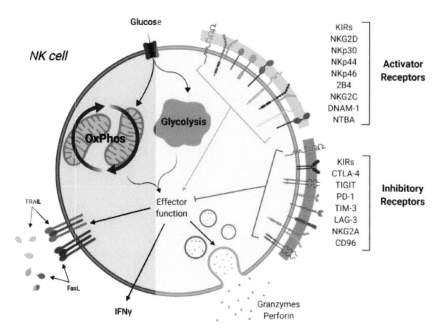

Figure-4: NK cell activation/inhibition. NK cells become activated through a complex network of activating receptors (green) and inhibitory receptors (red). Loss of inhibition or amplification of activating signals trigger NK cell activation, inducing metabolic changes and driving effector functions, including release of cytotoxic granules, pro-inflammatory cytokines (IFNγ), and death receptor signaling (TRAIL, FasL).

Credit: Fernández, Julián & Luddy, Kimberly & Harmon, Cathal & O'Farrelly, Cliona / International Journal of Molecular Sciences

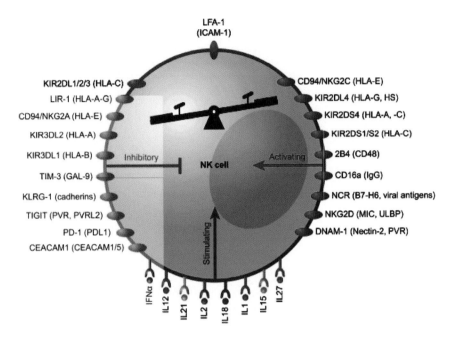

Figure-5: NK cell receptors, their function, and ligands. Schematic illustration showing how NK cell activity and cytotoxicity are controlled by signals from cell surface receptors. Cytokines and corresponding cytokine receptors on the NK cell are shown at the lower part of the NK cell. Inhibitory signals triggered by receptors (red) upon engagement of their ligands (in brackets) are shown on the left side of the NK cell. Activating signals triggered by receptors (green) upon engagement of their ligands (in brackets) are shown on the right side. Binding of LFA-1 (blue) on NK cells to ICAM-1 on target cells direct the granulae release toward the target cell, which is needed for efficient target cell lysis.

Credit: Carlsten, Mattias & Järås, Marcus / Frontiers in Immunology

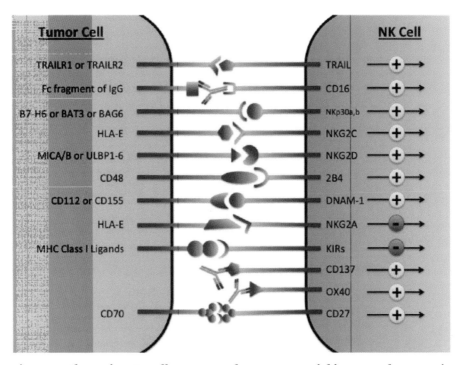

Figure-6: The major NK cell receptors that are potential immunotherapeutic targets. The transition of the NK cell from quiescence to activation is mediated by a network of activating and inhibitory receptors; it is the integration of the activating and inhibitory signals that determines if the NK cell becomes cytotoxic. Using immunotherapeutic agents to increase activation and decreases inhibitory signaling has the potential to generate NK cells with enhanced tumor lytic capacity.

Credit: Chester, Cariad & Fritsch, Katherine & Kohrt, Holbrook / Frontiers in Immunology

Inhibitory receptors play a crucial role in ensuring that NK cells do not accidentally activate against normal tissues - a mechanism referred to as "tolerance to self." For example, inhibitory KIRs (iKIRs) by human leukocyte antigen (HLA) class I molecules transmit an inhibitory signal to block NK cells triggering during effector responses. However, infected cells lack HLA class I molecules (a concept called "missing self"), which means NK cells will not receive any inhibitory signal.[8] Instead, cellular stress and DNA damage increase the regulation of "stress ligands," activating NK receptors and signaling the NK cell to kill the target.[8], [9]

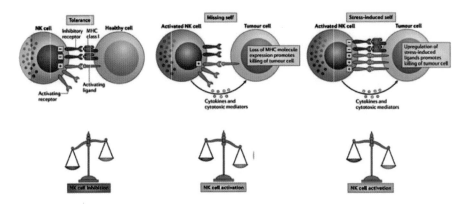

Figure-7: NK cell activation. The integration of inhibitory and activating receptors dictates the activation of NK cells. Ligation of inhibitory receptors to MHC class I on a healthy cell results in NK cell tolerance (left) whereas the NK cell becomes activated to kill a target cell as soon as MHC class I molecules are absent as for example on tumor cells (middle) or present at reduced levels (as it is typical for stressed cells) together with an overwhelming ligation of activating receptors. (Adapted and modified in arrangement from Vivier et al., 2012 105)

Credit: Hertwig, Laura / Humboldt University

There are various mechanisms of NK-mediated cytotoxicity. NK cells can directly kill tumor cells by releasing cytoplasmic granules containing perforin and granzyme, which prompt tumor cell lysis.[9],[10] Alternatively, NK cells can express tumor necrosis factor (TNF) family members like FasL and TNF-related apoptosis-inducing ligand (TRAIL), which induce tumor cell apoptosis by interacting with their respective receptors. Some NK cells contain the Fc receptor CD16 that induces degranulation against antibody-covered tumor cells, resulting in antibody-dependent cellular cytotoxicity (ADCC).[2]

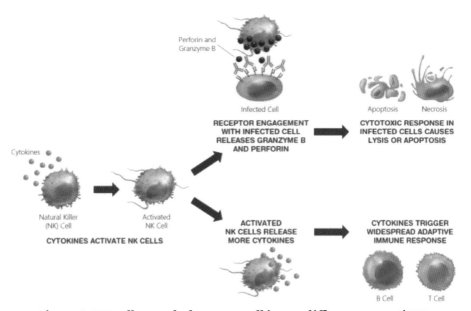

Figure-8: NK cells attack the target cell in two different ways. 1) NK cells attach directly to the target cell causing a cytotoxic chain reaction that destroys the cell. The NK cells release small cytoplasmic granules of proteins (perforin) and proteases (granzymes) that cause the target cell to die by apoptosis (programmed cell death). 2) NK cells also use another approach where they solicit help from other types of immune cells by releasing proteins in the blood (cytokines). These cytokines send signals out to the B cells and T cells triggering a more widespread immune response towards the target cells. The NK cells along with the other immune cells collectively attack and destroy the target cells.

Credit: NKMax Health

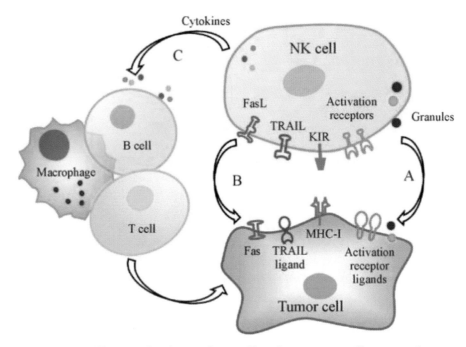

Figure-9: Killing mechanisms of NK cell against tumor cells. Upon the formation of immunological synapse between activated NK cell and tumor cell, multiple killing mechanisms can be triggered, including direct killing of the tumor cell by the (A) release of granules containing perforin and granzymes and (B) induction of apoptosis through the ligation of Fas-FasL or TRAIL-TRAIL ligand, and indirect killing through (C) the secretion of factors that recruit and promote the activation of other inflammatory cells that indirectly kill a target cell.

Credit: Fang, Fang & Xiao, Weihua & Tian, Zhigang / Frontiers of Medicine

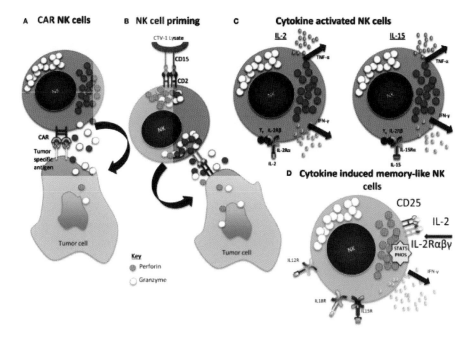

Figure-10: Summary of NK activation mechanisms. (A) CAR-NK cells. Expression of chimeric antigen receptor (CAR) specific for tumor-associated cell surface antigens redirects NK cells to malignant cells and facilitates cytotoxic activity. (B) Primed NK cells. Engagement of CD2 within CD15 of CTV-1 ligand leads to granule polarization and NK cell function is triggered by the engagement of at least one more activating receptor from a tumor cell. (C) Cytokine activated NK cells. IL-2 and IL-15 activation leads to activation of JAK/STAT, PI3K, MAPK, and NF-κB pathways. (D) CIML NK cells. IL-12, IL-15, and IL-18 induces a rapid and prolonged expression of CD25, resulting in a highly functional high-affinity IL-2 receptor. The receptor responds to picomolar concentrations of IL-2 leading to STAT5 phosphorylation and release of IFN-γ.

Credit: Domogala, Anna & Madrigal, J & Saudemont, Au / Frontiers in immunology

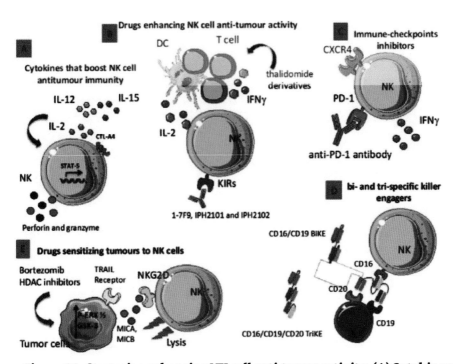

Figure-11: Strategies enhancing NK cell anti-tumor activity. (A) Cytokines such as IL-2, IL-15, and IL-12 alone or in combination can increase production and release of cytolytic granule content boosting NK cell anti-tumor immunity. (B) Drugs, including thalidomide derivatives, enhance the production of IFN-γ, thus triggering NK cell-mediated cytolysis. (C) Antibody directed to immune-checkpoints inhibitors like PD-1 can relieve the brake to NK cell cytolysis. (D) Bi-and tri-specific killer engagers strongly activate NK cell-mediated killing of tumor target cells. (E) Drugs able to sensitize tumors to upregulate ligands of activating receptors can increment killing of tumor cells; indeed, histone deacetylase inhibitors (HDAC) trigger the expression of NKG2DL such as MICA and MICB on tumor cells, these cells are more easily recognized and killed by NKG2D + NK cells.

Credit: Bassani, Barbara & Baci, Denisa & Gallazzi, Matteo & Poggi, Alessandro & Bruno, Antonino & Mortara, Lorenzo / Cancers

STRATEGIES TO INCREASE THE ANTI-TUMOR ACTIVITY

The ability of NK cells to exert rapid cytotoxicity against various hematologic malignancies including acute myeloid leukemia (AML),[11] ALL,[12],[13] multiple myeloma (MM),[14] as well as many solid tumors including neuroblastoma, ovarian, colon, renal cell, and gastric carcinomas make them suitable for use in adoptive therapy.[12],[15] However, different tumors have developed different evasion strategies to protect themselves from NK cells such as maintaining high surface expression of HLA molecules, becoming invisible,[13] or even lacking ligands that signal through activating NK cell receptors.

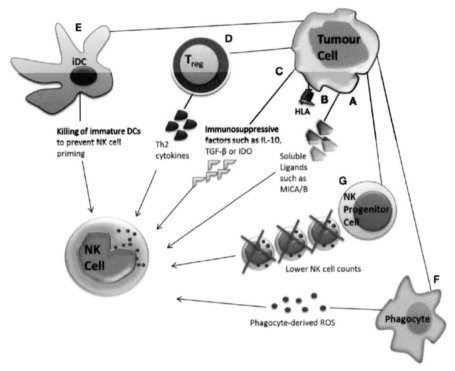

Figure-12: Tumor evasion strategies. Tumor cells can evade NK cell attack via direct or indirect mechanisms. Direct mechanisms include (A) shedding soluble ligands for NK cell activating receptors (B) upregulation of HLA molecules and (C) release of inhibitory cytokines. Indirect mechanisms
Credit: Sabry, May & Lowdell, Mark / Frontiers in immunology

Due to this, scientists have recently tried different strategies to enhance NK cell activity, one of which includes cytokines and artificial antigen-presenting cells (APCs) with enhanced costimulatory molecules as feeder cells for in vivo expansion. After incubation with cytokines, the NK cells gain the ability to kill tumors that are usually not sensitive to NK lysis. Scientists also use monoclonal antibodies (mAb) in combination therapy to boost ADCC.[16],[17],[18]

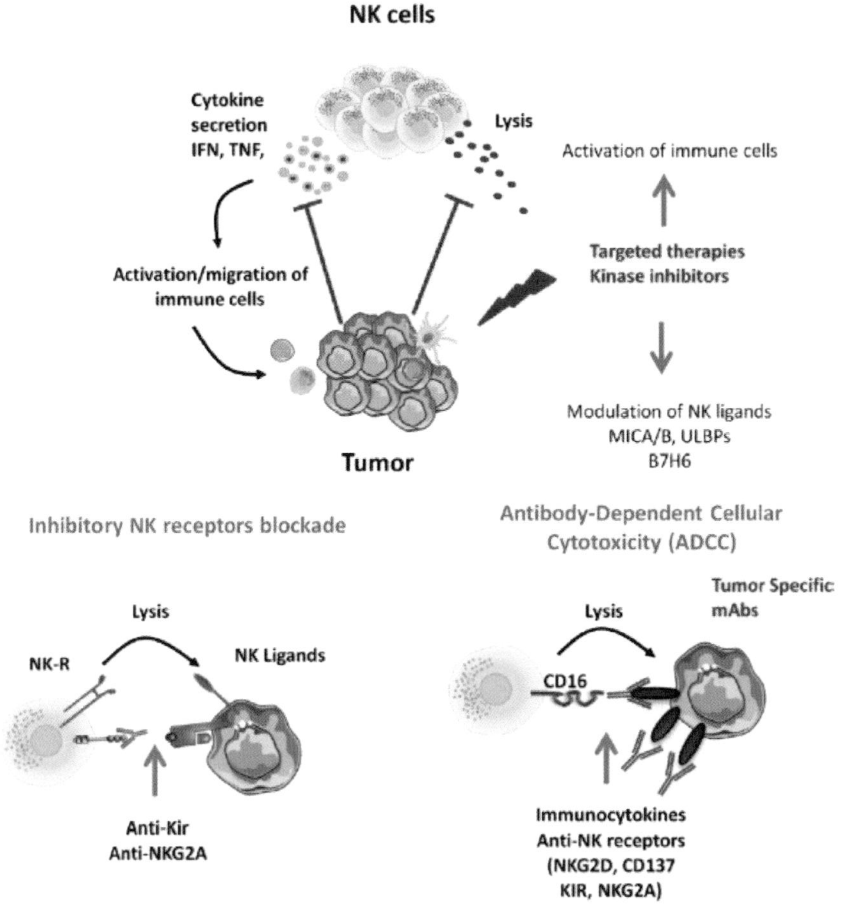

Figure-13: Natural killer (NK) cells infiltrating various tumor types display altered functions. Tumor-specific therapies may potentiate NK cell activation. Inhibitors targeting MAP kinase reduce tumor growth and display off-target effect modulating NK ligands expression and immune cell activation. Tumor-specific monoclonal antibodies (mAbs) may trigger ADCC by CD16 + NK cells. In that context, target NK-based immunotherapies may be proposed. Combined mitogen-activated protein kinase inhibitors with cytokines release NK function by inhibitory NK receptors [killer Ig-like receptor (KIR), NKG2A] blockade and promote NK-mediated ADCC of tumor antigen-specific mAbs and combined immunocytokines, anti-NK receptors (NKG2D, CD137, KIR, NKG2A).

Credit: Messaoudene, Meriem & Frazao, Alexandra & Gavlovsky, Pierre & Toubert, Antoine & Dulphy, Nicolas & Caignard, Anne / Frontiers in Immunology

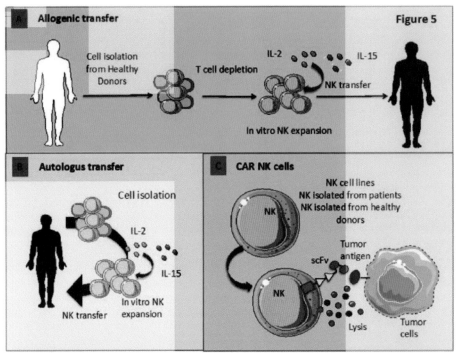

Figure-14: Strategies to increase the anti-tumor activity of adoptively transferred NK cells for anticancer therapy. (A) Allogeneic NK cells expanded ex vivo with IL-2 and/or IL-15 show a strong antitumor effect in patients which do not express the HLA-I allele recognized by inhibitory HLA-I receptors present on donor NK cells. (B) Also, autologous NK cells expanded ex vivo can be used to kill tumor cells. (C) Novel tools such as Chimeric Antigen Receptors (CAR) transduced into NK cells isolated from either healthy donors or patients can trigger transferred-NK cells to kill tumor cells. To avoid the variability of the NK cell activity from donor to donor, some NK cell lines have been transduced with CAR and used in clinical trials.

Credit: Bassani, Barbara & Baci, Denisa & Gallazzi, Matteo & Poggi, Alessandro & Bruno, Antonino & Mortara, Lorenzo / Cancers

In the past years, different groups of scientists have proven various methods of deriving functional NK cells for immunotherapy. Adoptive transfer of expanded, activated autologous NK cells, however, has not been very effective due to the inhibition of autologous NK cells by self-HLA molecules.[1],[15] Cells from an allogeneic source, on the other hand, have proven to be more promising for therapy. As seen in preclinical studies using adoptively transferred haploidentical NK cells, alloreactive NK cells can help create graft-versus-leukemia/tumor (GvL/GvT) effect without contributing to GVHD.[19],[20] Though the allogeneic NK cells are safe in patients with hematologic and solid tumors, they were only shown to be moderately effective in clinical activity.[4] Recently, scientists have been discussing new strategies to genetically reprogram the NK cells to enhance their cytotoxic ability, which primarily relies on redirecting NK cells by CARs (explained in the sections below).

CHALLENGES

Despite the many advantages of NK cells, there is hesitation to utilize NK cells for CAR-modified therapy. Since they have been restricted to pre-clinical trials, this questions their ability to migrate to and penetrate tumor tissues. Scientists are also rethinking the effects of the limited in vivo persistence of the NK cells because while it increases the safety of the treatment, it may reduce its effectiveness. Furthermore, although recent studies are proving to be more successful, there have been several impediments to the successful generation of CAR-NK cells for clinical use. In the past, genetic engineering of NK cells, even with viral methods, reported <10% transduction efficiency. The biggest challenge, however, is likely identifying appropriate target antigens that are pervasively expressed by tumor cells, but not expressed by normal tissue, thus limiting on-target off-tumor effects.

PRODUCING CAR NK CELLS

As explained above, there are many different ways to derive functional NK cells for adoptive therapy. All expanded, activated cord blood (CB), or peripheral blood (PB)-derived NK cells have their own capabilities that play an important role in gene modification. For example, expanded, activated NK cells are known for expressing many activating receptors like CD16, NKG2D, and NCRs. NK cells have also shown to reduce tumor activity in studies with hematologic malignancies such as AML. Furthermore, ex vivo NK cells produce a broader spectrum of cytokines including interferon (IFN)-γ, IL-3, and granulocyte macrophage colony-stimulating factor (GM-CSF), which is thought to reduce the risk of heart and kidney problems.

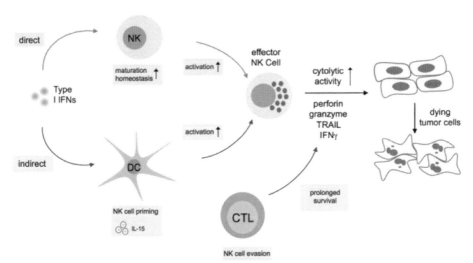

Figure-15: Interplay of type I interferons (IFNs) and natural killer (NK) cell activation during antitumor response. Type I IFNs either impact on maturation, homeostasis, and activation of NK cells, or indirectly influence NK cells to kill tumor cells via other immune cells or cells of the tumor microenvironment. Dendritic cells (DCs), in particular, are essential for NK cell priming via production of IL15. Another indirect effect of type I IFNs on NK cell function in cancer might result from modulation of surface molecules on CD8+ cytotoxic T lymphocytes (CTLs) [NCR1 ligands; classical and nonclassical major histocompatibility complex class I (MHC I)] leading to evasion of CTLs from NK cell-mediated elimination.

Credit: Müller, L., Aigner, P., & Stoiber, D / Frontiers in immunology

Most of the preclinical studies involving NK cells concentrated on targeting anti-CD19 and CD20-CARs in B cell malignancies.[21], [22] The infusion of CD19-CAR-T cells following lymphodepletion (destruction of lymphocytes and T cells) has shown to be very positive in cases where the patient has relapsed or refractory CD19+ malignancies. However, results have not been as positive for cases where the patient has refractory Burkitt lymphoma (BL). Scientists then began to target CD20+ aggressive B cell non-Hodgkin lymphoma using anti-CD20 CAR mRNA-modified expanded natural killer cells in vitro and in NSG mice. The anti-CD20-4-1BB-CD3ζ CAR was then used in the gene modification of PB NK cells from a group of healthy donors and was activated with a K-562-based feeder cell line that expressed membrane-bound IL-15 and 4-1BB ligand (K562-mbIL15-41BBL). After 16 hours, 50%–95% of the expanded PB NK cells expressed the CAR molecules, as well as an enhanced in vitro cytolytic activity against rituximab-sensitive and resistant BL cells. This also extended the survival of the Raji-xenografted mice.[23] However, in a clinical setting, these CAR molecules would likely need to be continuously infused several times due to its short-lived nature.

Nevertheless, a recent study has claimed to have found a new way to generate CAR-CD19+ NK cells that do not express the aforementioned limitation. The study genetically modified the CB-derived NK cell using a retroviral vector (iC9/CAR.19/IL15) with the gene for CAR CD19, allowing it to redirect specificity to CD19. The retroviral vector ectopically produced IL-15, a cytokine crucial for NK cell survival and proliferation, as well as expressed inducible caspase-9 (iC9), a suicide gene, that could be pharmacologically activated to eliminate transduced cells.[24] All of these features equipped the NK cells with the genetic modifications needed to competently kill the B cell leukemia or lymphoma cells.

It is important to understand the great variability in inherent NK cell functions between donors, the different methods used for gene modification, including viral and non-viral methods, and the various expansion strategies within the cells. Throughout the different studies done with NK cells (most of which utilize retrovirus- or lentivirus-based vectors), there has been a broad spectrum of transduction efficiencies with reports ranging from 1% to 90%.[21],[22] Lentiviral transduction is easily the most popular form of transduction because it has multiple benefits compared to retroviral transduction. For example, lentiviral transduction allows for the transduction of primary, non-activated cells since it does not need actively dividing cells. Nonetheless, scientists are exploring other non-viral transduction methods like electroporation, which immediately expresses the CAR molecule by introducing CAR-encoding mRNA through pores. However, due to the fact that mRNA electroporation and single lentiviral transduction usually result in lower PB and umbilical CB-derived NK cell efficiencies (<10% and <30% respectively in a study), retroviral transduction may be more appropriate for gene modification of primary and CB NK cells. One way to solve this problem would be to express the CAR in induced pluripotent stem cells (iPSCs) into mature NK cells, which will be explained in a later section.[25]

NK-92 CELLS

Most of the studies on NK cells have focused on the role of NK cell lines in the expression of CAR molecules, the most widely studied cell line being NK-92, a human cell line obtained from a non-Hodgkin's Lymphoma (NHL) patient. The specialty of NK-92 cells is that they are missing all inhibitory KIRs except KIR2DL4,[26] allowing in vitro activity against tumor targets. NK-92 cells have been administered in over 40 patients with advanced cancer. However, their efficacy is not sufficient even though they can be infused multiple times.[26] This has caused scientists to turn to CAR modification in hopes of increasing antitumor activity in the cells.

NK-92 cell lines, for various reasons, are theoretically thought to aid more positive results when genetically modified over primary NK cells. Firstly, NK-92 is a well-established cell line that has been reproduced and expanded repeatedly using good manufacturing practice (GMP)-compliant cryopreserved master cell banks and is plentiful for cancer therapy. Because of its potential, many scientists have genetically modified NK-92 cells to express CARs like CD19 and CD20, targeting hematologic and solid malignancies for B cell leukemia and lymphoma, CD38 and CS-1 for multiple myeloma, and HER-2 for epithelial cancers. Another specialty of NK-92 cells is that they can be given to patients through intratumoral injections, giving them the ability to traffic to tumor sites and produce a vaccine-like mechanism effect. Additionally, due to the uniformity of the cell line, NK-92 cells are more consistent with CAR expression with an average transduction efficiency of around 50%.[27],[28]

Although NK-92 cells have useful features like large-scale expansion and safety, they also have some disadvantages that need to be addressed. The most important drawbacks are that NK-92 cells are potentially tumorigenic (since they have to be obtained from a patient with NHL), express multiple cytogenetic abnormalities, and have latent infections with Epstein-Barr virus (EBV).[29] Therefore, to ensure safety, these cells are irradiated at minimum 1000 centrigrays (cGy) before clinical use, even though this reduces their in vivo proliferation, persistence, and long-term antitumor efficacy.[29] Moreover, though NK-92 cells can be repeatedly infused, continuous infusion may result in rapid rejection and cellular immunity against the allogeneic cell line.

NK CELL EXTRACTION FROM HUMAN PLURIPOTENT STEM CELLS

Another source where NK cells usable for CAR expression can be extracted from is human pluripotent stem cells (HPSCs) since both human embryonic stem cells (hESCs) and induced pluripotent stem cells (iPSCs) produce a limitless number of NK cells.

Lowe et al.[30] developed a strategy for the differentiation of NK cells from CD34+ human HPSCs isolated from cryopreserved CB, which were then modified to express CD19-CAR molecules. The study also described a platform to express other CAR molecules by using a feeder-free protocol for the generation of gene-modified NK cells from HPSCs using insulin-like growth factor 1.[30]

ACTIVATING NK CELLS

The CAR-NK constructs aforementioned all deal with the intra-cellular signaling chain CD3ζ, conferring specific cytotoxicity to surface-tumor antigens. An alternative strategy is developing CAR-NK cells that target ligands for activating NK receptors like NKG2D. The NKG2D ligands, major histocompatibility complex (MHC) class I chain-related A (MICA), MICB, and several UL-16-binding proteins (ULBPs) cover tumor and virally infected cells. This is why an NKG2D CAR can identify almost all (90%) human tumor types[31] and NKG2D ligands expressed on immunosup-pressive cells like myeloid-derived suppressor cells (MDSCs) and regulatory T cells (Tregs).[31]

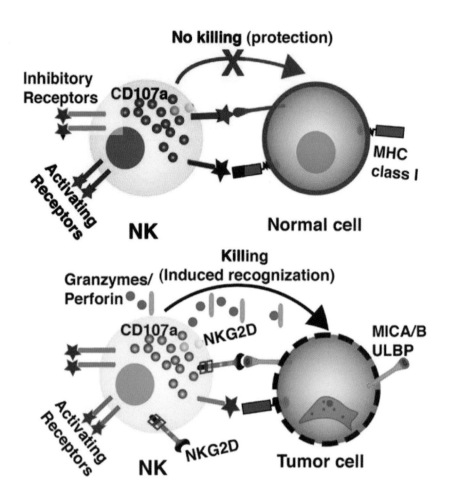

Figure-16: The interaction between NKG2D on NK cells and NKG2D ligands on tumor cells. In normal cells, NKG2D ligands express is very low. The functions of NK cells are balanced by the signals from the inhibitory and activating receptors. In humans, when normal cells are transformed into cancer cells. NKG2D ligands such as MICA/B and ULBP proteins, are often overexpressed. The engagement of NKG2D and NKG2D ligands overcomes inhibitory signals on NK cells, activates NK cells to release cytotoxic molecules such as perforin and granzyme, and trigger apoptosis of tumor cells.

Credit: Nayyar, Gaurav & Chu, Yaya & Cairo, Mitchell / Frontiers in Oncology

However, the ligands bring up the challenge of "on-target/off-tumor" toxicity as they are produced during physiological circumstances, such as inflammation. NKG2D CAR cells prompt enhanced cytotoxic activity because NKG2D cells lack signaling motifs. Moreover, the NKG2D CAR, when ligated, sends a signal via the phosphorylation of DNAX-activating protein 10 (DAP10), which in turn recruits downstream signaling effector molecules.[31] Cheng et al.[31] investigated if supraphysiologic activating signals (when there are above-average amounts of activating signals in the body) could enhance NK-mediated cytotoxicity. The study co-expressed DAP10 with the NKG2D/CD3ζ CAR and tested the activity of NK cells transduced with this CAR against multiple cell lines from various malignancies. Intriguingly, there were positive responses with all the cell lines, including osteosarcoma, prostate carcinoma, and rhabdomyosarcoma. However, this strategy resulted in the loss of activating ligands on few primary hematologic malignancies, ultimately affecting NKG2D-mediated cytotoxicity. Surprisingly, no correlation was found between the level of NKG2D ligand expression and NKG2D-DAP10-CD3ζ receptor-mediated cytotoxicity.

Topfer et al.[32] wanted to identify a CAR that could activate NK cells using a different method. The study incorporated DNAX-activation protein 12 (DAP12) and prostate stem cell antigen (PSCA) scFv (derived from the hybridoma 7F5) in primary NK cells and the NK cell line YTS. While DAP12 is expressed in NK cells (as is in many activating receptors), the anti-PSCA-DAP12 CAR is expressed in primary NK cells as well as the YTS-NK cell line. It also has the ability to lyse otherwise resistant PSCA+ HLA-B/C- and HLA-C-matched tumor cells. Interestingly, the anti-PSCA-CD3ζ-based CAR did not enhance cytotoxicity as well as the YTS-NK CAR incorporating the DAP-12 signaling domain. This finding was crucial; to this date, it is the first to show that a single immunoreceptor tyrosine-based activation motif (ITAM)-containing DAP12-CAR can signal as effectively as a CD3ζ-based CAR containing three ITAMs. Furthermore, this DAP12-signaling CAR did not need any extra costimulatory signaling molecules for in vitro activation and cytotoxicity.

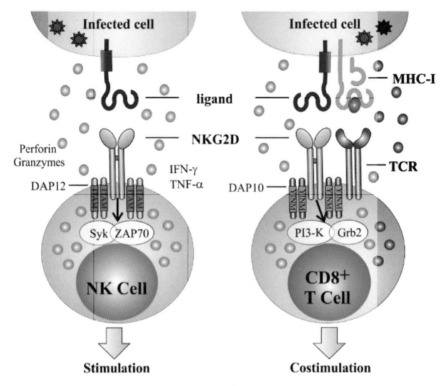

Figure-17: NKG2D acts as an activating and a co-stimulatory receptor. NKG2D is a type-2 transmembrane homodimer that signals via association with adapter molecules DAP10 or DAP12. Association with DAP12 leads to phosphorylation of the ITAM and triggering of the Syk and/or Zap70 signaling cascade. Association with DAP10 results in tyrosine phosphorylation on the YINM motif and recruitment of the PI3K and Grb2 cascade. On NK cells, NKG2D serves as an activation receptor, such that NKG2D engagement is sufficient to trigger NK cell-mediated cytotoxicity and cytokine production. In contrast, NKG2D acts as a co-stimulatory receptor on CD8 T cells, requiring TCR-mediated signaling for their full activation. Grb2, growth factor receptor-bound protein 2; IFN-γ, interferon γ; ITAM, immunoreceptor tyrosine-based activating motif; PI3K, phosphoinositide 3-kinase; Syk, spleen tyrosine kinase; TCR, T cell receptor; TNF-α, tumor necrosis factor α; Zap70, zeta-chain associated protein kinase 70.

Credit: Slavuljica, Irena & Krmpotić, Astrid & Jonjic, Stipan / Frontiers in immunology

While CAR modification is an effective immunotherapy, engineered NK cells can also increase cell cytotoxicity by expressing cytokines. This strategy might be even more beneficial than CAR modification as it increases NK cell persistence whilst eliminating the need for a toxic in vivo cytokine supplementation. However, a major challenge is overcoming the risk of inducing CRS, cytokine-induced systemic toxicity, and malignant transformation in the transduced cells. Some scientists have proposed the idea of temporarily introducing genes coding for IL-2 or IL-15 using short-lived expression models like mRNA electroporation to avoid toxicities.

IS CAR-NK CELL THERAPY READY FOR CLINICAL USE?

Though there have been clear positive results with both CAR-NK cells and CAR-T cells, as well as a strong safety profile for non-genetically modified NK cells, there have only been two clinical trials of CAR-NK cell therapy with patients (NCT00995137 from St. Jude Children's Research Hospital and NCT01974479 from The National University Health System, Singapore). The trials are using an identical second-generation anti-CD19 CAR with the 4-1BB costimulatory domain (anti-CD19-BB-ζ) to target refractory CD19+ ALL.[33] Though the Singapore trial is open to all ages, the St. Jude trial was limited to pediatric patients and is no longer accepting patients. This dose-escalation trial gives patients a single intravenous (i.v.) infusion of anti-CD19-BB-ζ NK cells at doses of 0.5×10^7 to 1×10^8 CD56+ cells/kg. Clinical results are still being awaited.

In the last year, more studies regarding CAR-NK cell therapy were conducted and registered on ClinicalTrials.gov. One example is PersonGen BioTherapeutics, which was given permission to administer sequential doses of third-generation (relevant scFv attached to TCRζ, CD28, and 4-1BB signaling domains) CAR-transduced NK-92 cells (on days 0, 3, and 5). The study is focusing on targeting refractory CD7+ leukemia and lymphoma in adults (NCT02742727), CD33+ myeloid malignancies in children and adults (NCT02944162), refractory CD19+ ALL malignancies in patients undergoing hematopoietic stem cell transplantation (HSCT) (NCT02892695), and MUC1+ relapsed and refractory solid tumors (NCT02839954). Other scientists are working to determine the safety and efficacy levels of escalating doses of off-the-shelf CB-derived NK cells, which express iC9.CAR19.CD28-ζ-2A-IL-15 for relapsed or refractory B-lymphoid malignancies.

Undoubtedly, several challenges and questions must be answered before CAR-NK therapy can be used to treat more patients. Though many trials have explained strategies for isolation, expansion, and transduction of NK cells, the generation of the cells is still long and difficult. While retroviral constructs have greater efficacy than lentiviral constructs, they have a greater risk of contributing to the development of insertional mutagenesis (the phenomenon by which an exogenous DNA sequence integrates within the genome of a host organism), creating a regulatory hurdle. Insertional mutagenesis may also result in the deregulation of genes close to the insertion site and can potentially cause cellular transformation if it induces the deregulation of oncogenes or tumor suppressor genes. In order to avoid the risks of oncogene activation and insertional mutagenesis, several scientists have used electroporation. Unfortunately, the trials reported a very low success rate, with transfection efficiencies as low as 10%.[27] Transfection of DNA and mRNA into several immune type cells was successfully reported by Rabinovich et al.[40] using the Amaxa Nucleofector system. However, due to certain intrinsic properties of NK cells (some being more amenable to non-physical transfection modalities), this system did not improve transfection efficiency in this trial. Additionally, since CAR molecule expression usually lasts less than 7 days, it is likely to lower the long-term efficacy level of the CAR-NK cells.[34]

Another question that still needs to be studied is whether the infused allogeneic CAR-NK cells will be rejected and if so, whether lymphodepletion will be necessary. The problem is that lymphodepleting chemotherapy will deplete other immunosuppressive cells within the tumor-like Tregs and MDSCs, which will hurt NK cell cytotoxicity and in vivo expansion. Due to some of the safety questions raised with infused CAR-modified T cells, scientists are looking into whether a suicide system (e.g. based on caspase-9 or thymidine kinase) or programmed cell death, will need to be incorporated.[24],[35],[36]

Despite the several preclinical trials done following CAR-NK and CAR-T cells, there are still many unanswered questions such as whether repeated infusions could trigger immunogenicity, elicit human anti-mouse antibodies (HAMAs) or cause cellular-mediated rejection/sensitization in CAR-NK cells. The question of HAMA immunogenicity has been explored in CAR-T cells and has proven not to be a concern. This is likely as many of the patients have received a single infusion of autologous cells.

In order to establish a safe and effective CAR-NK immunotherapy, further studies regarding the optimal vector, construct, and transduction method are crucial.

PROMISE OF NK CELLS IN IMMUNOTHERAPY

We are in an exciting era in the field of cellular therapy and many new ideas for cancer treatment are being explored. The theory of NK cell immunotherapy is one of the most promising strategies against refractory malignancies due to its high cytotoxicity. NK cells have proven to be significantly more diverse than originally thought and have shown great potential in tumor control and immunosurveillance. Most importantly, NK cells hold great promise for the development of an off-the-shelf cellular product that could eliminate the need for a patient-specific diagnosis and could be readily available for immediate clinical use. Although much has been discovered, there are still a number of questions that must be addressed before NK cells can be extended to larger cohorts of patients. For example, it is very important to identify the ideal vector, signaling endodomain, and costimulatory molecule for NK cells that will be most effective and safe. In order to do this, different combinatorial techniques will have to be tested to improve the efficacy of tumor-specific NK cells. This will likely be done by harnessing the innate power of the NK cell, inhibiting or knocking out immune checkpoints, or by targeting the tumor microenvironment. Furthermore, additional gene-editing techniques like CRISPR/Cas9 and transcription activator-like effector nuclease (TALEN) will have to be analyzed in the setting of NK cells. Currently, only one clinical trial recruiting patients is exploring this strategy,[37],[38],[39] although trials targeting NY-ESO1 and PD-1 are in development. Without a doubt, therapeutic strategies designed to leverage engineered NK cells will make a significant contribution to the development of emerging cancer treatment strategies.

CONCLUSION

Recently, cellular therapies have focused primarily on genetic-ally engineered chimeric antigen receptor (CAR) autologous T cells to identify tumor antigens. Though CD19-redirected T cell therapy for B-lymphoid malignancies has shown positive re-sults, the generation of autologous products for each patient is challenging, expensive, and logistically unreasonable in the long run. Additionally, allogeneic T cells carry a significant risk of GVHD mediated through their native T cell receptor whilst NK cells constitute a valuable, safe and versatile allogeneic product for immunotherapy. Unlike T cells, NK cells do not need prior antigen sensitization to mediate cytotoxicity. NK cell cytotox-icity is mediated primarily through degranulation and antibody-dependent cellular cytotoxicity (ADCC), mediated by CD16 bind-ing to the Fc portion of IgG1 opsonized on the surface of target cells. Since NK cells do not require time to develop an immune response, they are useful in instant cell-targeted killing. Further-more, the safety of NK cells as demonstrated in their efficacy in human trials in the allogeneic setting expands possible sources of NK cell therapy beyond just autologous products. Given advances in genetic engineering, it is likely that CAR-engineered NK cells will contribute to new immunotherapeutic approaches for treat-ment against refractory hematological malignancies.

Table 1. Table comparing the advantages and disadvantages of CAR-T cell therapy and CAR-NK cell therapy.

CAR-T Cell Therapy	CAR-NK Cell Therapy

Advantages:
The use of CAR-T cell therapy reduces the need for aggressive chemotherapy. As a result, patients have a shortened recovery period than after stem cell transplants with aggressive chemotherapy.

CAR-T cells have shown to achieve remission rates that last for years. CAR-T cell therapy has even been effective in patients whose cancer returned after several other treatments.

Advantages:
NK cells are able to mediate cellular cytotoxicity against cancer cells without the risk of inducing GVHD.

Allogeneic NK cells hold great promise for the development of an off-the-shelf cellular product that could eliminate the need for a patient-specific diagnosis and could be readily available for immediate clinical use.

CAR-NK cells provide greater immunosurveillance when compared to CAR-T cells because they retain their full array of native receptors that can recognize and target tumor cells. Even if the CAR target antigen is downregulated, the CAR-NK cells will still be able to attack tumor cells more effectively than CAR-T cells. This results in increased chances of survival and lower chances of relapse in patients receiving NK cell therapy.

NK cells have shorter lifespans than T cells, allowing them to quickly die after mediating cytotoxicity and reducing long-term effects such as prolonged cytopenia caused by on-target/off-tumor toxicity to normal tissues.

Disadvantages:	Disadvantages:
The generation of a patient-derived autologous CAR-T cell product is too cumbersome and restrictive for widespread clinical use. Manufacturing time for CAR-T cells takes a minimum of two to three weeks, making it an impractical choice for patients with rapidly advancing disease. CAR-T cell therapy involves the transportation of allogeneic T cells from a donor, which increases the risk of GVHD, where the donor T cells will attack the healthy host cells. GVHD can occur any time after transplant and can range from mild to severe, though most cases are life-threatening.	Though it has not yet been confirmed, the shorter life-span of NK cells may reduce their efficacy following adoptive transfer.

REFERENCES

[1] Locatelli F., Moretta F., Brescia L., Merli P. Natural killer cells in the treatment of high-risk leukemia. *Semin. Immunol,* (2014): 26:173–179.

[2] Farag S.S., Caligiuri M.A. Human natural killer cell development and biology. *Blood Rev,* (2006): 20:123–137.

[3] Moretta L., Locatelli F., Pende D., Marcenaro E., Mingari M.C., Moretta A. Killer Ig-like receptor-mediated control of natural killer cell alloreactivity in haploidentical hematopoietic stem cell transplantation. *Blood,* (2011): 117:764–771.

[4] Yoon S.R., Lee Y.S., Yang S.H., Ahn K.H., Lee J.H., Lee J.H., Kim D.Y., Kang Y.A., Jeon M., Seol M. Generation of donor natural killer cells from CD34(+) progenitor cells and subsequent infusion after HLA-mismatched allogeneic hematopoietic cell transplantation: a feasibility study. *Bone Marrow Transplant,* (2010): 45:1038–1046.

[5] Sotillo E., Barrett D.M., Black K.L., Bagashev A., Oldridge D., Wu G., Sussman R., Lanauze C., Ruella M., Gazzara M.R. Convergence of acquired mutations and alternative splicing of CD19 enables resistance to CART-19 immunotherapy. *Cancer Discov,* (2015): 5:1282–1295.

[6] Campbell J.J., Qin S., Unutmaz D., Soler D., Murphy K.E., Hodge M.R., Wu L., Butcher E.C. Unique subpopulations of CD56+ NK and NK-T peripheral blood lymphocytes identified by chemokine receptor expression repertoire. *J. Immunol,* (2001): 166:6477–6482.

[7] De Maria A., Bozzano F., Cantoni C., Moretta L. Revisiting human natural killer cell subset function revealed cytolytic CD56(dim)CD16+ NK cells as rapid producers of abundant IFN-gamma on activation. *Proc. Natl. Acad. Sci. USA*, (2011): 108:728–732.

[8] Campbell K.S., Hasegawa J. Natural killer cell biology: an update and future directions. *J. Allergy Clin. Immunol*, (2013): 132:536–544.

[9] Bradley M., Zeytun A., Rafi-Janajreh A., Nagarkatti P.S., Nagarkatti M. Role of spontaneous and interleukin-2-induced natural killer cell activity in the cytotoxicity and rejection of Fas1 and Fas-tumor cells. *Blood*, (1998): 92:4248–4255.

[10] Screpanti V., Wallin R.P., Ljunggren H.G., Grandien A. A central role for death receptor-mediated apoptosis in the rejection of tumors by NK cells. *J. Immunol*, (2001): 167:2068–2073.

[11] Stringaris K., Sekine T., Khoder A., Alsuliman A., Razzaghi B., Sargeant R., Pavlu J., Brisley G., de Lavallade H., Sarvaria A. Leukemia-induced phenotypic and functional defects in natural killer cells predict failure to achieve remission in acute myeloid leukemia. *Haematologica*, (2013): 99:836–847.

[12] Bachanova V., Miller J.S. NK cells in therapy of cancer. *Crit. Rev. Oncog*, (2014): 19:133–141.

[13] Rouce R.H., Shaim H., Sekine T., Weber G., Ballard B., Ku S., Barese C., Murali V., Wu M.F., Liu H. The TGF-β/SMAD pathway is an important mechanism for NK cell immune evasion in childhood B-acute lymphoblastic leukemia. *Leukemia*, (2016): 30:800–811.

[14] Swift B.E., Williams B.A., Kosaka Y., Wang X.H., Medin J.A., Viswanathan S., Martinez-Lopez J., Keating A. Natural killer cell lines preferentially kill clonogenic multiple myeloma cells and

decrease myeloma engraftment in a bioluminescent xenograft mouse model. *Haematologica*, (2012): 97:1020–1028.

[15] Gras Navarro A., Björklund A.T., Chekenya M. Therapeutic potential and challenges of natural killer cells in treatment of solid tumors. *Front. Immunol*, (2015): 6:202.

[16] Romain G., Senyukov V., Rey-Villamizar N., Merouane A., Kelton W., Liadi I., Mahendra A., Charab W., Georgiou G., Roysam B. Antibody Fc engineering improves frequency and promotes kinetic boosting of serial killing mediated by NK cells. *Blood*, (2014): 124:3241–3249.

[17] Kanazawa T., Hiramatsu Y., Iwata S., Siddiquey M., Sato Y., Suzuki M., Ito Y., Goshima F., Murata T., Kimura H. Anti-CCR4 monoclonal antibody mogamulizumab for the treatment of EBV-associated T- and NK-cell lymphoproliferative diseases. *Clin. Cancer Res*, (2014): 20:5075–5084.

[18] Lin W., Voskens C.J., Zhang X., Schindler D.G., Wood A., Burch E., Wei Y., Chen L., Tian G., Tamada K. Fc-dependent expression of CD137 on human NK cells: insights into "agonistic" effects of anti-CD137 monoclonal antibodies. *Blood*, (2008): 112:699–707.

[19] Ruggeri L., Capanni M., Urbani E., Perruccio K., Shlomchik W.D., Tosti A., Posati S., Rogaia D., Frassoni F., Aversa F. Effectiveness of donor natural killer cell alloreactivity in mismatched hematopoietic transplants. *Science*, (2002): 295:2097–2100.

[20] Olson J.A., Leveson-Gower D.B., Gill S., Baker J., Beilhack A., Negrin R.S. NK cells mediate reduction of GVHD by inhibiting activated, alloreactive T cells while retaining GVT effects. *Blood*, (2010): 115 4293–4230.

[21] Imai C., Iwamoto S., Campana D. Genetic modification of primary natural killer cells overcomes inhibitory signals and induces specific killing of leukemic cells. *Blood*, (2005): 106:376–

383.

[22] Li L., Liu L.N., Feller S., Allen C., Shivakumar R., Fratantoni J., Wolfraim L.A., Fujisaki H., Campana D., Chopas N. Expression of chimeric antigen receptors in natural killer cells with a regulatory-compliant non-viral method. *Cancer Gene Ther,* (2010): 17:147–154.

[23] Chu Y., Hochberg J., Yahr A., Ayello J., van de Ven C., Barth M., Czuczman M., Cairo M.S. Targeting CD20+ aggressive B-cell non-Hodgkin lymphoma by anti-CD20 CAR mRNA-modified expanded natural killer cells in vitro and in NSG mice. *Cancer Immunol. Res,* (2015): 3:333–344.

[24] Di Stasi A., Tey S.K., Dotti G., Fujita Y., Kennedy-Nasser A., Martinez C., Straathof K., Liu E., Durett A.G., Grilley B. Inducible apoptosis as a safety switch for adoptive cell therapy. *N. Engl. J. Med,* (2011): 365:1673–1683.

[25] Hermanson D.L., Kaufman D.S. Utilizing chimeric antigen receptors to direct natural killer cell activity. *Front. Immunol,* (2015): 6:195.

[26] Tonn T., Schwabe D., Klingemann H.G., Becker S., Esser R., Koehl U., Suttorp M., Seifried E., Ottmann O.G., Bug G. Treatment of patients with advanced cancer with the natural killer cell line NK-92. *Cytotherapy,* (2013): 15:1563–1570.

[27] Boissel L., Betancur M., Wels W.S., Tuncer H., Klingemann H. Transfection with mRNA for CD19 specific chimeric antigen receptor restores NK cell mediated killing of CLL cells. *Leuk. Res,* (2009): 33:1255–1259.

[28] Boissel L., Betancur-Boissel M., Lu W., Krause D.S., Van Etten R.A., Wels W.S., Klingemann H. Retargeting NK-92 cells by means of CD19- and CD20-specific chimeric antigen receptors compares favorably with antibody-dependent cellular cytotoxicity. *Onco-*

Immunology, (2013): 2:e26527.

[29] Uphoff C.C., Denkmann S.A., Steube K.G., Drexler H.G. Detection of EBV, HBV, HCV, HIV-1, HTLV-I and -II, and SMRV in human and other primate cell lines. *J. Biomed. Biotechnol,* (2010): 2010:904767.

[30] Lowe E., Truscott L.C., De Oliveira S.N. In vitro generation of human NK cells expressing chimeric antigen receptor through differentiation of gene-modified hematopoietic stem cells. *Methods Mol. Biol,* (2016): 1441:241–251.

[31] Chang Y.H., Connolly J., Shimasaki N., Mimura K., Kono K., Campana D. A chimeric receptor with NKG2D specificity enhances natural killer cell activation and killing of tumor cells. *Cancer Res,* (2013): 73:1777–1786.

[32] Töpfer K., Cartellieri M., Michen S., Wiedemuth R., Müller N., Lindemann D., Bachmann M., Füssel M., Schackert G., Temme A. DAP12-based activating chimeric antigen receptor for NK cell tumor immunotherapy. *J. Immunol,* (2015): 194:3201–3212.

[33] Shimasaki N., Fujisaki H., Cho D., Masselli M., Lockey T., Eldridge P., Leung W., Campana D. A clinically adaptable method to enhance the cytotoxicity of natural killer cells against B-cell malignancies. *Cytotherapy,* (2012): 14:830–840.

[34] Zhao Y., Moon E., Carpenito C., Paulos C.M., Liu X., Brennan A.L., Chew A., Carroll R.G., Scholler J., Levine B.L. Multiple injections of electroporated autologous T cells expressing a chimeric antigen receptor mediate regression of human disseminated tumor. *Cancer Res,* (2010): 70:9053–9061.

[35] Zhou X., Dotti G., Krance R.A., Martinez C.A., Naik S., Kamble R.T., Durett A.G., Dakhova O., Savoldo B., Di Stasi A. Inducible caspase-9 suicide gene controls adverse effects from alloreplete T cells after haploidentical stem cell transplantation. *Blood,*

(2015): 125:4103–4113.

[36] Rouce R.H., Sharma S., Huynh M., Heslop H.E. Recent advances in T-cell immunotherapy for haematological malignancies. *Br. J. Haematol*, (2017): 176:688–704.

[37] Poirot L., Philip B., Schiffer-Mannioui C., Le Clerre D., Chion-Sotinel I., Derniame S., Potrel P., Bas C., Lemaire L., Galetto R. Multiplex genome-edited T-cell manufacturing platform for "off-the-shelf" adoptive T-cell immunotherapies. *Cancer Res*, (2015): 75:3853–3864.

[38] Qasim W., Zhan H., Samarasinghe S., Adams S., Amrolia P., Stafford S., Butler K., Rivat C., Wright G., Somana K. Molecular remission of infant B-ALL after infusion of universal TALEN gene-edited CAR T cells. *Sci. Transl. Med*, (2017): 9:eaaj2013.

[39] Qasim W., Amrolia P.J., Samarasinghe S., Ghorashian S., Zhan H., Stafford S., Butler K., Ahsan G., Gilmour K., Adams S. First clinical application of Talen engineered universal CAR19 T cells in B-ALL. *Blood*, (2015): 126:2046.

[40] Rabinovich P.M., Komarovskaya M.E., Ye Z.J., Imai C., Campana D., Bahceci E., et al: Synthetic messenger RNA as a tool for gene therapy. *Hum Gene Ther*, (2006); 17: pp. 1027-1035

PHOTO CREDITS

Cover Image: Niaid. (2016, August 25). Human Natural Killer Cell. Retrieved from https://www.flickr.com/photos/niaid/29228845335/

Figure-1: Cancer Research UK. Diagram showing how cancer cells keep on reproducing to form a tumor CRUK 127.svg. (n.d.). Retrieved from https://commons.wikimedia.org/w/index.php?curid=34333362

Figure-2: Hucks, George & Rheingold, Susan. (2019). The journey to CAR T cell therapy: the pediatric and young adult experience with relapsed or refractory B-ALL. Blood Cancer Journal. 9. 10.1038/s41408-018-0164-6.

Figure-3: Niaid. (2016, August 25). Human Natural Killer Cell. Retrieved from https://www.flickr.com/photos/niaid/29228845335/

Figure-4: Fernández, Julián & Luddy, Kimberly & Harmon, Cathal & O'Farrelly, Cliona. (2019). Hepatic Tumor Microenvironments and Effects on NK Cell Phenotype and Function. International Journal of Molecular Sciences. 20. 4131. 10.3390/ijms20174131.

Figure-5: Carlsten, Mattias & Järås, Marcus. (2019). Natural Killer Cells in Myeloid Malignancies: Immune Surveillance, NK Cell Dysfunction, and Pharmacological Opportunities to Bolster the Endogenous NK Cells. Frontiers in Immunology. 10. 2357. 10.3389/fimmu.2019.02357.

Figure-6: Chester, Cariad & Fritsch, Katherine & Kohrt, Holbrook. (2015). Natural Killer Cell Immunomodulation: Targeting Activating, Inhibitory, and Co-stimulatory Receptor Signaling for Cancer Immunotherapy. Frontiers in Immunology. 6. 10.3389/fimmu.2015.00601.

Figure-7: Hertwig, Laura. (2016). The implication of natural killer cells and neutrophils in autoimmune disorders of the central nervous system. 10.18452/17591

Figure-8: Natural Killer Cells. (n.d.). Retrieved from https://nk-maxhealth.com/natural-killer-cells/

Figure-9: Fang, Fang & Xiao, Weihua & Tian, Zhigang. (2018). Challenges of NK cell-based immunotherapy in the new era. Frontiers of Medicine. 12. 10.1007/s11684-018-0653-9.

Figure-10: Domogala, Anna & Madrigal, J & Saudemont, Au. (2015). Natural Killer Cell Immunotherapy: From Bench to Bedside. Frontiers in immunology. 6. 264. 10.3389/fimmu.2015.00264.

Figure-11: Bassani, Barbara & Baci, Denisa & Gallazzi, Matteo & Poggi, Alessandro & Bruno, Antonino & Mortara, Lorenzo. (2019). Natural Killer Cells as Key Players of Tumor Progression and Angiogenesis: Old and Novel Tools to Divert Their Pro-Tumor Activities into Potent Anti-Tumor Effects. Cancers. 11. 461. 10.3390/cancers11040461.

Figure-12: Sabry, May & Lowdell, Mark. (2013). Tumor-Primed NK Cells: Waiting for the Green Light. Frontiers in immunology. 4. 408. 10.3389/fimmu.2013.00408

Figure-13: Messaoudene, Meriem & Frazao, Alexandra & Gavlovsky, Pierre & Toubert, Antoine & Dulphy, Nicolas & Caignard, Anne. (2017). Patient's Natural Killer Cells in the Era of Targeted Therapies: Role for Tumor Killers. Frontiers in Immunology. 8. 10.3389/fimmu.2017.00683.

Figure-14: Bassani, Barbara & Baci, Denisa & Gallazzi, Matteo &

Poggi, Alessandro & Bruno, Antonino & Mortara, Lorenzo. (2019). Natural Killer Cells as Key Players of Tumor Progression and Angiogenesis: Old and Novel Tools to Divert Their Pro-Tumor Activities into Potent Anti-Tumor Effects. Cancers. 11. 461. 10.3390/cancers11040461.

Figure-15: Müller, L., Aigner, P., & Stoiber, D. (2017). Type I Interferons and Natural Killer Cell Regulation in Cancer. Frontiers in immunology, 8, 304. https://doi.org/10.3389/fimmu.2017.00304

Figure-16: Nayyar, Gaurav & Chu, Yaya & Cairo, Mitchell. (2019). Overcoming Resistance to Natural Killer Cell Based Immunotherapies for Solid Tumors. Frontiers in Oncology. 9. 10.3389/fonc.2019.00051.

Figure-17: Slavuljica, Irena & Krmpotić, Astrid & Jonjic, Stipan. (2011). Manipulation of NKG2D Ligands by Cytomegaloviruses: Impact on Innate and Adaptive Immune Response. Frontiers in immunology. 2. 85. 10.3389/fimmu.2011.00085.

ABOUT THE AUTHOR

Priyanka Senthil

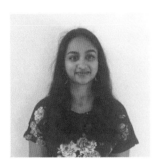

Priyanka Senthil is a high school student in Reno, Nevada. Currently, she is working with mice expressing the parvalbumin gene, with the goal of understanding the molecular and cellular mechanisms underlying neural plasticity. Some of her previous research experiences include studying the newly discovered Calyx of Held in hopes to learn more about synaptic signaling. Priyanka also worked at the Center for Genomic Medicine, Massachusetts General Hospital, researching cerebral small vessel disease and intracerebral hemorrhage risk among different ethnic groups.

WORKS BY THIS AUTHOR

BRAIN: The Most Complex Organ

This book provides an introduction to neuroscience for young students. Topics discussed include: the nervous system, neurotransmitters and receptors, action potentials and synaptic transmission, early brain development, somatosensory systems, neurodegenerative disorders, brain imaging techniques, and brain machine interfaces. This book aims to inspire future scientists, doctors, and researchers by explaining fundamental concepts in neuroscience in a way that is easy to understand by audiences of all ages. The book explores how the brain works, how we think, how we perceive the world, and the neural mechanisms that underlie devastating degenerative diseases like Alzheimer's, Parkinson's, Multiple Sclerosis, and Huntington's, among others. Recently, several novel methods for sequencing the human genome and genetic engineering have been developed, enabling better visualization and stimulation of nerve cells and connections in the brain. This book highlights these rapid advances and provides readers with a succinct but comprehensive discussion of the field of neuroscience.

View on Amazon:
https://www.amazon.com/dp/B08DSVC95F/

NeuralFit

NeuralFit is an app that helps patients with Alzheimer's and any dementia-related symptoms by reducing the rate of cognitive decline through quick and engaging brain-training games. The app includes research-backed games that fall into one of the following categories: speed, concentration, memory, attention, and advanced skills. One of the games asks players to memorize a grocery list in the order it is presented to track their memory capabilities. Another game challenges players to dodge obstacles on the road to test the speed of their brain signaling/processing and to improve their reaction time. Another game asks players to identify the incorrectly spelled word among a list of 10 words within a given time limit to increase players' processing ability. Our games hope to stimulate players' brains and keep their brains active and challenged even throughout adulthood to ensure efficient neural functioning and communication. Our game also has a feature to track players' progress to show them how they have been progressing. The app is being used in a study to evaluate differences in cognitive performance among elderly individuals in different countries. The study also seeks to evaluate differences in cognitive improvement as a result of continuous daily training with the app. The current results of our study show that young adults who engaged in brain training games demonstrated improvements in brain processing speed, working memory, and executive functions. And it is not only young adults who might benefit from brain training. Similar research studies agree with our current findings that older adults who take part in 1-hour brain training sessions for 10 days over a 5-week period are less likely to develop cognitive decline or dementia. NeuralFit can be found on the Google Play Store as a free download for all who are interested. Check it out for yourself!

Download from Google Play Store:
https://play.gogle.com/store/apps/details?
id=com.PriyankaSenthil.NeuralFit

Printed in Great Britain
by Amazon

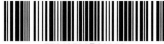

77640586R00038